Recovering from Mental Illness for Clients and Caregivers

Brian Catanzaro, MA

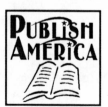

PublishAmerica
Baltimore

First printing

ISBN: 1-4241-6158-4
PUBLISHED BY PUBLISHAMERICA, LLLP
www.publishamerica.com
Baltimore

Printed in the United States of America

Dedicated to all clients and caregivers stricken with mental illness who are searching for a path to comfort and joy.

I would like to thank the Creator of the Universe for the ability to write this book and for the answer to prayers; Dr. Sanjeevani Jain for her suggestion to tell my story and giving me the inspiration to help others with this book; to colleagues, friends, and clients I have worked with throughout the years, and my family for their support through dark times.

Contents

The statements in this book are not intended to replace advice given by medical and mental health care professionals. Mental illness can be dangerous and life-threatening if not treated with the guidance of a psychiatrist and mental health care professionals. Every individual case requires specialized individual treatment based on the client's life experiences and physical and mental health.

Suggestions for treatment made in this book may not be appropriate for all clients. This book is also designed to be useful information for family or significant other care-givers.

Ideas presented in this book should be used only after consulting with the client's psychiatrist, counselor, and physician, and the client has monitoring and support systems available for use as part of on-going treatment.

Preface
My Story: Relapse and Recovery

First Hospitalization

I began psychotherapy on the advice of a friend, who suggested that I had a lot of "emotional baggage." She thought that medication might help me also. I became anxious in and out of therapy sessions. I developed the delusion that the police would arrest me for past wrongdoings. During one session I became extremely anxious and the counselors suggested that I try medication to help me calm down. They stated that I could be admitted to the hospital in-patient Psychiatric ward and could get medication. I went to Psychiatric Emergency Services, was screened and voluntarily admitted for being psychotic. I was diagnosed as a schizophrenic and prescribed Thorazine. My mother helped me to pay accumulating bills and rent and I was able to keep my apartment and personal belongings, otherwise I would have lost all of my property. Loss of all personal property occurs frequently for people who become psychotic and require a hospital stay.

I needed to attend a group for aftercare and in order to see a psychiatrist for prescriptions. I attended the only group available at night, which was at a hospital located one hour away from my apartment. I didn't like Thorazine because it made me sleepy and took away my sex drive. I didn't like being called a schizophrenic because I was able to hold a job, pay my bills, go to college at night and play music in a band. I found a doctor of alternative medicine whose previous practice was psychiatry and went to him seeking to be treated without using Thorazine or other drugs. I did not want to take drugs for the rest of my life. I did not want to live with the side effects.

Meanwhile I was able to finish up an associates degree in humanities/ art at the local community college. Medication helped to make this possible, but I didn't see that side of the story.

Second Hospitalization

I stopped using medication when I fell in love with a singer. We lived together for seven months and I was truly happy and did not feel psychotic. When my girlfriend decided that she didn't want to be married I couldn't bear the loss. Living alone, I eventually became delusional again and decided to try and get admitted to a hospital. I was admitted and diagnosed as having schizoaffective disorder and was prescribed a different medication, which I don't recall. I do recall being allergic to Haldol. It causes me to shake, shiver, and convulse. So I have had bad experiences with medication. However, I went back to the alternative doctor who prescribed the antipsychotic Navane. I loved Navane. I felt no side effects from it. Life was improving. I gave up my apartment to move to the university campus to complete my undergrad degree. I alternated from living on campus to living with my mother and sister. I earned a BA in Music Therapy and completed a five-year program in three years with the help of my transfer credits. Again I did not realize that medication was making it possible to cope with and achieve lifetime accomplishments.

Third Hospitalization

I thought everything was going pretty well but the doctor informed me that Navane had irreversible side effects with long-term use and I would eventually have to stop taking it. I had gotten a new apartment and had a steady job and began to take graduate courses and work toward an MA. The doctor suggested Risperdal. I became very dizzy on Risperdal and could not function. I decided to go without medication. I couldn't handle pressures at my job and quit. I was going broke and began to look for a job. I returned to the Catholic Church and still believe in Christianity today. My faith helped me to cope with life's pressures. I had become psychotic and knew it. I tried to get admitted to the local state hospital but they refused to admit me.

I decided on a whim to go to a counseling center. I got into an argument with some counselors about learning disabilities and was taken away by the police after raising my voice to the counselors. I agreed to be admitted voluntarily to a hospital that I had been in the first time, years ago. If I had refused to be admitted voluntarily they were ready and had the power to commit me involuntarily.

During the hospital stay I continued to argue with counselors and demanded to be seen by psychiatrists. I refused meds until seeing the doctors. I began to take a newer antipsychotic called Zyprexa. The doctor told me right to my face, " You're bipolar, it's a disease and the treatment is medication." I had already lost my apartment, but thanks again to my mother, my belongings were placed in storage. The movers stole my coin collection and a few other valuables, but I could have lost everything without my mother's help. I was close to defaulting on my car loan payment and it was only through the mercy of the doctors that I was spared that financial hardship. I began to use the hospital outpatient services for medication and monitoring by a doctor.

Almost all of my hospital expenses were covered by state-funded Charity Care because I had very little income. The first hospital stay went into collections and I had to pay several thousand dollars to a collection agency, which was a very unpleasant experience. However, the bulk of that bill was covered by some kind of low-income funding program.

Eventually I got my old job back and was able to get student loans and an apartment and finish graduate school. I stopped using the alternative doctor. I was able to change jobs to better working conditions and finished the MA in counseling. I now realize from working in the field of group home counseling and from personal experience that the right medication can create recovery from mental illness. I know that without medication I become manic, disoriented, easily confused, and anxious. Medication stops the mania and allows me to accomplish life tasks and responsibilities. I now see a psychiatrist in town for medication monitoring. I liked Zyprexa, but it has been shown to cause diabetes and weight gain, so I currently am taking a combination of drugs for stabilization. I also believe that faith in Christianity saved me from evil environments and consequences.

Today I am a group home counselor, volunteer as a DJ at the local college radio station, perform music in restaurants and coffee houses and participate in church activities. Marriage is an objective.

Developmental Stages of Recovery

Stage I: The Client Becomes Aware of Mental Illness and Treatment

1. Remission and Recovery

Remission is the successful treatment of symptoms. Treatment is successful when symptoms are abated, happen less frequently, or completely stop. For example you may stop hearing voices inside your head. You may stop feeling depressed and begin to laugh at humorous things. You may stop feeling hyper and are now able to focus your attention for longer periods of time on something of interest instead of wanting to run away. In order to strive for remission, you need to get as much information about your illness as you can. You can ask your psychiatrist what your symptoms are. Some doctors are reluctant to talk about symptoms of mental illness to those who are not in the field. This brings up the issue of diagnosis. If symptoms change over time or medication is not effective in reducing symptoms, your diagnosis may be changed. A diagnosis is generally used as a summation of a case or a reference term for other mental health professionals. Some doctors do not like to talk about diagnosis because they don't want to put a permanent label on someone. They also don't want a person to convince themself that they have a certain illness and "act out" behaviors that they think they should. Diagnosis may change later on, but if you have been hospitalized for psychosis, or dangerous or extreme behavior, a psychiatrist will be able to identify a set of symptoms which you are presenting. You should try to speak to the doctor about which symptoms she or he would like to see reduced. Then you will be able to report back with more meaningful information when she asks you how you are doing. You can also ask the doctor how you are doing in order to get some clinical feedback and some idea of behaviors or life goals to strive for. You can also ask your counselor to discuss your illness and identify some of its symptoms. Your counselor may be able to direct you to some reading material about your illness or medications.

Recovery is an on-going process. Once psychotic symptoms are in remission you can begin to think about how you want to live your life. The abatement of symptoms clears up the psychotic part of your personality so that you now may be able to accomplish things you only dreamt about in the past. Some examples of this are making new friends, going to college, taking music lessons, working toward getting your own apartment, or writing a book.

The first step to recovery is accepting the fact that you have a mental illness and that you need to take medication in order to maintain your best mental health. As one doctor stated:

"It's a disease, you have it, and the treatment is medication every day." In order to live your life in a healthy, successful way, you must take the responsibility of complying with treatment.

There is also another challenge, however, to consider during recovery. New medications enter the market every few years or sooner. These new medications may be more effective for some people and may have less side-effects. Your psychiatrist may want to try a new med to eliminate harmful side-effects from your current med. If a doctor thinks it is in your best interest to try a new med, you've got to accept that she is trying to help you. You may not feel any different on the new med. If your symptoms start to return, you can tell your doctor. It is helpful to attend any "Medication Education" groups or to read information about your medications. Keep in mind that you may also have to live with some side-effects. The most common side-effect is drowsiness. You can ask the doctor if you can take your meds before bedtime. You would be amazed at how less drowsy you may feel during the daytime after doing this. Part of recovery is accepting the fact that you may be drowsy sometimes. This drowsiness may prevent you from driving a car, so you would have to consider public transportation as an alternative. There are public transportation programs throughout the community that are available to the disabled and payable through disability benefits in your state. Another way to combat drowsiness is by drinking coffee. However caffeine can reduce the effectiveness of your meds so don't drink it all day long or else your symptoms may return. Any counselor, nurse, or doctor will tell you that. You have to live with side-effects but you may not have them severely enough to make you disabled. Don't give up!

What Can Happen If You Don't—Critical Thinking Skills Exercise

You might wake up one day feeling great. You may think that you are cured and you no longer need to take medication and get that drowsy feeling. You must challenge this thought with the opposite thought. That is, you are feeling great because the medication is working and you need to continue taking it to continue feeling great. If you do not take your medication you are taking a big risk: the risk that your behavior could cause you to be committed to a hospital stay. Then you would be back to "square one" and have to start all over again to re-earn some of the freedoms and benefits of being out of the hospital.

2. Relapse and Hospitalization

Relapse occurs when psychotic symptoms return. Such symptoms include hallucinations, hearing voices, or becoming so anxious or depressed that you cannot perform every day activities, losing your sense of time, becoming disoriented and other signs of becoming unable to get through the day without assistance. Relapse can lead to inappropriate behaviors which can cause you to be brought to a hospital for treatment by your family, friends, police, or someone in the community. If you do return to the hospital, your goal would then become to get out of the hospital and into a treatment program. This is usually called a "Discharge Plan." In order to achieve the goal of being out, you must comply with your treatment while in the hospital. The staff and doctors need to know that you are making an effort to get well by following their instructions. Compliance in the hospital includes taking the medication, attending all meals, attending to personal hygiene, which is regular showering, shampooing and shaving, doing your laundry and keeping your room neat by making the bed. You may not be eligible for recreation, but you can ask to attend. An entire book can be devoted to wellness during a psychiatric hospital stay, but if you have been there before you will have a better idea of what to do in order to obtain a discharge plan and discuss discharge with the doctors and nurses who are treating you. You may make friends while you are in the hospital, but it is not likely that you will continue to see them afterwards, that is, it would take a great effort to do so and people often return to their previous social groups and neighborhoods which will be unfamiliar to you. If you are a Christian, you may be able to obtain a Bible and can meditate on scripture to help you cope. Sometimes

Catholic clergy or lay ministers visit and administer the Sacraments. If you are of the same ethnic or cultural background as one of the staff, you may be able to find some common ground for discussion with the staff if they are not busy, or a doctor or nurse who is treating you. You will be continuously observed and expected to show "positive" behaviors, or behaviors that indicate that your symptoms are being reduced and that you are making an effort to get well.

What Can Happen If You Don't—Critical Thinking Skills Exercise

If you refuse to take your medication or do not show signs of sedation, you will be watched more closely to see if you are taking your medication. If you do not take it you may be restrained and given medication by force. You will have been given many chances to take it on your own before this can happen. If you do not eat regularly you may become malnourished, or your thinking processes may be hindered. You may wish to request a certain type of meal, such as meatless or low calorie meals, if that is what you are used to. If you refuse to attend activities on the ward it will be recorded and you will be watched even more closely than before. The less you comply, the longer you will remain on the ward and the further away from a discharge plan you will be. If you do nothing to help yourself you may be sent to a long-term care hospital to live semi-permanently, or until you are placed in a group home. You could lose your possessions and will need to learn how to live in the world of a hospital, far away from Main Street, USA.

3. Life After the Hospital and Basic Needs

Your hospital stay eventually comes to an end and you are given and accept the responsibility for your discharge plan. You are now in charge of your medical and psychiatric care. When you return home you can begin to concentrate on your basic needs. Basic needs include obtaining a psychiatrist, transportation, a healthy diet, outpatient psychotherapy, a physician for general health, a safe environment, and finding out about income benefits.

Many hospitals offer outpatient services. They may include group therapy sessions, which can help you educate yourself about your illness. Outpatient services can also help you maintain visits and care from a psychiatrist. You must inquire about where these meetings are held and which doctor is available for you to see. You need to find out about income so you can continue to pay for and receive medications. If you are going back to work you need to find a psychiatrist who is in your insurance network. The most immediate needs are resuming an income and obtaining medication. You also need to find out about getting transportation so you can get to your medical appointments and continue seeing the psychiatrist. You may be able to see a psychiatrist as an outpatient at the same hospital. Psychotherapy groups may also be available on an outpatient basis.

Take advantage of these opportunities. It is then time to set up your income. Your local Social Services and Social Security offices can inform you of Disability Income eligibility, (SSD or SSI,) and may be able to help you obtain transportation from community-based companies who provide rides to medical appointments for the disabled. If you are fortunate enough to be able to live with family, perhaps family members can assist you in keeping your appointments. If you were unable to keep your job, you must then accept help from state and local charity organizations. Psychotherapy can be done on an individual basis, that is one-on-one with a therapist, or can be obtained in group therapy. Groups can help you to network with others who have been in the hospital. You are not alone. Groups can also provide helpful community resources that can help you receive the care that you need. Once your income and medical insurance is decided upon it is easy to register with outpatient services, a pharmacy and even transport service companies. Group or individual counselors can help you to learn how to obtain and manage your needs. The immediate goal is to obtain the services you need to remain stable on medication and to obtain psychiatric care. If you live at home, many of these arrangements and appointments can be made by phone. The sooner these needs are met, the sooner you can consider returning to work. If you decide that you cannot work or have become disabled you then need to rely on your family members for assistance. If you do not have family to lean on then you are homeless and will likely not be discharged to the community, but to a long-term care hospital. Once you are in long-term care your only recourse is to wait and request application to a group home. It will take time for an opening to come up for a group home. Unfortunately, while you are waiting, you are subject to the rules of the long-term care hospital. If you show compliance and behavior that demonstrates that you are willing and trying to get better, your chances of being considered for discharge can only increase. Psychiatry, psychotherapy and education are the keys to wellness. You may also have spiritual or religious beliefs. If you do, then you may inquire about religious services, clergy or ministers who may provide services to your facility.

Developmental Stages of Recovery

Stage II: The Client Begins to Work with Professionals in the Mental Health System

4. Life in a Group Home

The goals for living in a group home are similar to those of living in a hospital. You need to be compliant with taking medication, seeing a psychiatrist and general practice doctors, keeping your room and yourself clean, and staying safe by following the rules. The rules are in place to help you get well and possibly move to more independent living status. Group homes vary in the amount of staff supervision needed to run them. Level A status is given to a home where staff is on site 24 hours and day, 7 days a week. The people that are cared for are not referred to as "patients," but as "clients" or "consumers," since they require on-going care and are consumers of mental health services. Staff members assist clients in all activities of daily living, or ADLs. Those activities include obtaining medical services, providing transportation, recreational activities, counseling, managing finances, keeping house, and getting along with your housemates. Clients who can accomplish ADLs with the minimum of supervision are described as "higher-functioning" clients. Those who need more supervision to accomplish ADLs are described as "lower-functioning" clients. Usually, house meetings are held to keep everyone aware of the rules and what is expected from clients and staff in order to give everyone the care they need. Keep in mind that staff are trained in the care of others and usually attend training meetings during work hours to keep up with the current practices in the field and the community. Level B and C group homes and apartments are visited by staff weekly and clients are provided with services as needed. In order to achieve more independence and move to less-supervised housing you must show that you are coping with your transition, are compliant with the rules and work with staff instead of working against them. The staff and the agency who provide group home services are responsible for your well-being and strive to provide safety for you and your housemates.

What Can Happen If You Don't—Critical Thinking Skills Exercise

If you break the rules, chances are that privileges will be taken away from you, such as recreation trips, rides to places you enjoy going to and increasing the amount of chores you will be required to perform. If you do not make an effort to get along with housemates and staff you take the risk that you will be evicted from the group home, which means you may return to a hospital setting. If you have any problems while living in a group home you should discuss them with staff. Usually you will have a specified staff member working on your case. Sometimes they are called "your one-to-one." Problems and discomforts should be discussed with your one-to-one case manager in order to find ways of coping while observing the rules of the group home, the community and your medical and psychiatric treatment. If spirituality is a significant activity in your life you can work with your case manager in order to find ways of observing your beliefs that will be compatible with group home activities. Your one-to-one can be consulted if you like to shop at a particular store. If you have family that you regularly visit with, arrangements can be made for overnight visits and packing your medications by consulting your case manager. Instead of ignoring the rules, you can work toward independence by communicating with staff. Another example of this is having the desire to work at a part-time job. However, you need to know that the amount of money you are able to earn may be restricted by requirements for obtaining social security benefits. Therefore your working hours may be limited to one or two days per week. Generally speaking, if you follow the rules you will achieve your goals sooner.

5. Boundaries and Working with Staff

It is likely that you will find your case manager or case worker to be helpful, as long as you have been following the rules of the group home. A case manager or one-to-one counselor is not your friend, however. Group home staff are people who enjoy helping others, but this relationship is not to be mistaken for a friendship. Staff are not provided for you to engage in a love relationship either. Staff will not become your boyfriend or girlfriend. These are the boundaries. A boundary is the distance between you and staff, or other service providers. You would not expect to become friends with a doctor or nurse. It is the same with staff. They are providing services to you. If you are grateful for the help, saying thank you is enough. You may also desire to purchase gifts for staff, but this is usually not permitted. Staff are often not permitted to accept gifts for their services. Providing services is what they are paid to do, and is included in clients' rent. Staff are not there to become intimately involved with you or other clients. You should not expect to become a "favorite" of staff. If you follow the rules and complete your ADLs, you will be considered by the treatment team of staff and clinician as to whether you are ready to attempt new responsibilities and privileges. The goal of living in the group home is to begin to return to the community. Staff are like nurses, who are providing a service. Many of the services provided by a case manager are paid for by state benefits that you are entitled to receive for being medically needy, disabled, or receiving a very low income. Staff can help you to keep informed of the rules of the agency and group home.

Every Level A group home with 24/ 7 supervision will have a staff office. If you need staff you are expected to go to their office to request help. Calling out for staff by yelling across the house is not the appropriate way of contacting staff, unless it is an emergency and a case of serious injury where you are unable to walk to the office. Staff are not butlers or maids called on to run at your beck and call. You need to knock on the office door. Staff may be busy at that time and will arrange to meet you at a specified time in order to assist you with your questions or needs. You are also required to clean up after yourself. Staff may remind you to clear your place at the table if you have left dirty dishes behind. You may also be responsible for your household chores, such as vacuuming, preparing dishes for the dishwasher or preparing dinner. Staff are there to do it with you, not do it for you.

Here is an example of working with your one-to-one. Staff may ask you to clean your room of unnecessary items. If you have no where to put them, staff might suggest that you purchase a shelf unit to help organize your belongings. Your case manager will be able to obtain money for the purchase from your benefits and, if necessary, make a withdrawal from your bank. You can then go shopping for a unit with your one-to-one and they can help you to assemble it. Then you are responsible for making use of it and keeping your room uncluttered. Staff and house rules may require you to throw away unusable items that are causing clutter in your room.

The hope is that you will be able to become less reliant on staff as time goes on, and that you will begin to function independently with less help from staff. You can work toward this goal at your own pace, with assistance from staff. Be prepared to do your chores, attend house meetings, clean up after yourself, report for your medication at the specified time, keep medical appointments, budget your money, and other tasks on your own, and not wait for staff to tell you. You have the power to take the first step in completing your responsibilities in the group home. You don't have to wait to be told to do things. Try to learn what is expected of you as a member of the household and take steps on your own to complete the tasks you are responsible for. Furthermore, it will make life easier if you remember to treat your housemates with courtesy and respect, as you would staff, doctors and nurses who provide personal needs care to you.

It is not a good idea to measure your progress by what other clients have achieved. You will observe that some of your housemates are not able to do many things without the help of staff. You yourself may find that you need more help from staff than others. Every case is different. All you can do is your best. You are not required to help the others complete their responsibilities. That is why staff are there.

6. Working Toward Independent Living

If you observe the rules, make peace with your client peers, and don't take your opportunities for granted, you may become eligible to move to the next level and get an apartment by yourself or with fewer roommates. That means that staff will still be available to you, but they will not be there 24 hours, 7 days per week. It means you may be able to work part-time, or even full-time, depending on your rent, disability benefits, and safety and medical needs. You will also have the opportunity to make new friends and network with peers to find out about community activities that you can attend. These activities can include recreation, work, volunteering, going to college or even going to church. Working with staff and complying with your medical treatment needs are the ways of reaching your goals sooner than later. Communication with staff, even in less-supervised housing, remains an important key in the process of achieving independence.

What Can Happen If You Don't—Critical Thinking Skills Exercise
Remember what your alternatives are if you don't follow the rules. The reality is you have gone from the hospital to being homeless. If it weren't for working with staff and your current agency you could end up back in a hospital. That means losing all of the privileges you have become used to. If you don't take your medication without direction from your psychiatrist, you will be on a one-way road to a relapse in psychosis. That means you will become further mentally ill and require treatment in a hospital setting until you become stable again. Further, that means that you will lose contact with the agency you are currently working with and have to wait for a future opening with a completely

different social and medical community. You may have to start over by living in a Level A group home with an unknown group of people, thereby losing friends you have made as well. You can lose all of the progress you have made and your goal of independence will become a shattered dream.

Developmental Stages of Recovery

Stage III: The Client Attempts to Maintain Good Mental Health and Well-Being

7. Living with Family

Depending on your age and living situation, living with family can be arranged as part of a discharge plan. For someone in their 20s or 30s, returning home to parents may be helpful. Someone older may not wish to live with a parent or parents. In that case they can be referred to a group home agency and apply to live there. A parent or parents who take in an adult child being discharged from the hospital may not be aware of the complex basic needs of a person requiring psychiatric care. Many of the basic needs were listed in the previous chapter. They include obtaining a psychiatrist, transportation, a healthy diet, outpatient psychotherapy, a physician for general health, a safe environment, and financial arrangements for income benefits. A parent or guardian would have to educate themself on how to obtain these basic services from all of the outside agencies involved, such as the Social Security Office. One of the advantages of living in a group home is that staff and management of the group home agency are already trained on how to obtain these services. A parent may not be aware of how to obtain financial benefits which pay for medication and it would take longer for a client to receive medication at a reduce cost, potentially causing a very large bill to accumulate. Obtaining medication benefits is one of the highest priority tasks because medications can be very costly, some 50 dollars per pill or more. A parent may also be unaware of the various day programs that may be available to clients or which ones would be most appropriate for their adult child. Attendance in a day program can help a client to learn how to cope with living in the community and can offer group and individual psychotherapy for the client. Such programs can also provide education about medication and mental illness to clients. Some day programs may provide transportation, otherwise the parent would have to arrange for transport from another agency that specializes in it. In other words, communicating and coordinating a number of outside services is essential and most beneficial for a client in order to learn about how to return to and function in the community while coping with their illness. The issue of boundaries also exists within a family. The client may not become more independent by relying on their parent to coordinate their care. When possible, it is in the client's best interest to learn how to provide outside care for themselves, or a client may become too dependent on the parent or guardian and miss opportunities for living independently in the community. Not all clients are capable of living by themselves in the community. In that case, the great burden of 24 hour care falls on the parent or guardian. It may not be possible to maintain the level of care needed 24 hours a day by one or two parents or guardians. An agency is best at providing this level of care because they have a greater amount of staff. The chances for a relapse or crisis increases in a family setting due to a lack of supervision or the inability to provide urgent care or crisis intervention. A parent or guardian may not recognize the need to call 911 or may be hesitant in the case of a behavioral crisis incident, which can place the client at further risk of the consequences of relapse.

8. Obtaining Services

The living situations of individuals may vary, but whether you are taking care of yourself, have been discharged to a group home, or are living with family, a comprehensive approach to basic needs and mental and physical health services is necessary for on-going care and to prevent relapse. A person that can participate in many social functions easily is said to be "higher-functioning." A person who is able to participate in fewer functions on their own and needs to be directed frequently is said to be "lower-functioning." We all have physical, emotional and social needs. Some of these needs can be satisfied by our families and some can be obtained from outside agencies. A person with a mental illness will need the following:

Housing and rental assistance
A psychiatrist
A medical doctor for general health care
Financial assistance and management
Counseling
Recreation among peers and the community
Transportation
Spiritual and Philosophical support

Housing and Rental Assistance

Following a hospital stay in an acute care psychiatric unit, the hospital needs to know that the client will have a place to sleep and be protected from the elements. That environment will also observe a medication regimen and other medical needs of the client. There are several options for discharge. One is living with family members who are able to allow the client to live with them, two is a return to a long-term care psychiatric hospital. The third is for senior clients, which is discharge to a long term care psychiatric nursing home. Fourth is to a group home agency who has agreed to accept the client and allows the client room and board in one of their homes.

Living with family is a challenge to family members and the client because they need to make sure that the client takes medication daily and are able to attend to other medical needs of the client, as well as provide room and board. Money for housing assistance may be available from the state, however the family may not know how to apply for it. Also, the family will need to provide transportation for the client for medical, social and recreational activities. These are just a couple of issues that demonstrate the burden of taking care of a family member with mental illness. Not all families know where to find the resources that can help to ease the financial and environmental burden of caring for a client 24 hours a day, 7 days per week. When a client lives in a group home, staff are trained to apply for and acquire financial, medical, and transportation assistance for clients. These include rental assistance from the state and social security or disability income from the federal government. The client's rent pays for all of the services provided by the group home, including room and board. Living in a group home makes a client eligible for various financial assistance programs, whereas living with family may not meet some eligibility requirements. In some states, a family member may elect to become a guardian of the client. Becoming a guardian opens up opportunities for receiving housing assistance and other financial benefits, however it is a greater time commitment for the guardian to be able to act in place of the client. In a group home setting, a client is given the opportunity, when possible, to make decisions about their health care and become empowered for working toward more independent living in the future. If a client has a guardian, the client is not able to manage some of their affairs.

Psychiatrist

A psychiatrist is trained specifically in the methods of using medication to reduce the symptoms of mental illness. A general practice doctor can write prescriptions for any medicines, but they do not have the training in psychiatric care. A psychiatrist is a necessary component in a client's treatment plan in order to help him or her maintain activities of daily living and to prevent relapse. Psychiatric treatment is included in group home care. When a client lives with family, there is a chance that psychiatric care may be disrupted. A client may refuse to see a doctor, and this may lead to a behavioral crisis incident, or a "breakdown." If a crisis exists, a family member may be resistant to calling the police for help. If a client refuses to see a doctor in a group home setting he or she runs the risk of eviction and returning to a long-term care psychiatric facility. If a client has a behavioral crisis incident in a group home he or she may be committed to a hospital for psychiatric evaluation in order to determine if they need to be placed under acute care. In this way, their treatment is uninterrupted. In a family environment, a crisis may occur and the opportunity for psychiatric treatment may be missed. This is important because sometimes medication doses need to be adjusted in order to reduce symptoms that are indicated by behavior changes. If a client has been refusing or not swallowing their medication, symptoms can return. Some psychotropic medications, such as Clozaril or Depakote, require monthly blood testing to monitor physical changes and prevent toxic reactions. A client needs to see a psychiatrist at least once per month, or more frequently, and must comply with a psychotropic medication schedule in order to remain stable and safe from potential symptoms and crisis.

Medical

Older clients will need more medical care than younger clients. In a family setting, medical issues may be overlooked. Some of them are allergies, skin care, care for chronic injuries, such as bone or muscle injuries, weight control, diabetes, and foot care. Clients who are overweight may not be able to reach down in order to take care of their feet. Diabetes needs to be managed, as well as other diseases, for example Lyme disease, high cholesterol, or thyroid irregularities. Again this is an additional burden on family members and medical issues may go undetected. A group home setting is more beneficial for clients because it includes timely annual physicals. Visits with a general practice doctor can be easily made whenever a client has a discomfort that may place them at-risk for poor health.

Financial Assistance and Management

Many financial benefits are available from state and federal government for care of the chronically ill, and that includes mental illness. Some of them are Medicare, state programs for the medically needy, (In New Jersey it is called Medicaid,) state rental assistance, Social Security, Social Security Disability Benefits, and there may be other state programs that assist with living expenses, such as heating and cooling assistance for a resident or tenant. Agencies are very experienced with obtaining these benefits and managing the living expenses of clients. For inexperienced family care-givers, a considerable amount of time and effort will be required to educate themselves about available benefits and to apply for them. For example, some applications have annual or quarterly deadlines and some programs are for temporary assistance. Applying for and obtaining financial benefits for clients is something that a group home agency does on a daily basis.

Counseling

Counseling is helping someone who is troubled by guiding them toward new insights. A counselor does not tell someone what to do, but helps them determine what their options are for changing thoughts, behaviors and their environment. Encountering the symptoms of mental illness or emotional breakdown or trauma or stress requires a period of time for stabilization and distance from a world of confusion. After that distance is experienced and stability occurs, the client can return to a world of confidence. During that time of distance is when counseling is most needed. A client leaving behind a period of extreme emotional stress needs guidance in order to learn and resume functioning for daily living.

A family member can act as a counselor by directing the client to complete tasks of every day living. Counselors in group homes also provide this service. The family member and the group home counselor need to perform in a similar way, that is by structuring the daily routine of activities for a client. That structure is a planned schedule of activities that occur at the same time every day, week, or month. Here is an example: Breakfast is at 7 a.m., Medications are at 7:30 a.m., Day Program is at 9 a.m., Dinner is at 5 p.m., Shopping trip is at 6 p.m., Medications are at 7 p.m., and so on. On Saturdays is a trip to the mall. On Sundays some clients are driven to church and picked up later. Monday night is movie night, Tuesday is visitor's night, Saturday and Sunday may be reserved for clients who go on family visits, et cetera. The activities are structured. This helps a person to know what to expect and removes uncertainty in their life. Structured activities are an emotional safety zone. The certainty of structure replaces the uncertainty of emotional trauma. The client gains assurance that he or she will experience something comfortable and familiar when following the structure. Every minute of life does not need to be structured. There are times when optional activities will present themselves or a vacation with family can be planned and coordinated by the team of doctor and counselors. In a group home, counselors will direct clients, that is tell them what needs to be done in order to keep the structure of safety and comfort intact. The client is free to refuse or to give input for changing the activity. A client refusing to cooperate with the structure runs the risk of unhealthy living conditions and possible eviction. For example, a client who's turn it is to make dinner refuses to wash her hands. She must be redirected or not allowed to cook that day. In a group home, clients are assigned treatment plans, which are the basis of structured activities.

Group home counselors meet with and help clients talk through difficulties and experiences. This may be more difficult for a solitary family care-giver. In a 24/7 group home there are several counselors always present who can address issues as they occur. Since most family members need to work or go to school, there may be only one person to guide the client, which is more stressful for the care-giver.

Recreation

A person recovering from a crisis due to mental illness is able to participate in community activities that are enjoyable. Clients like to go to movies, go shopping and meet with friends. Their friends, or peers, may also suffer from mental illness and it is helpful for peers to meet and share their experiences. Peers sharing experiences helps a person to measure progress they have made and acknowledge that they are safe, as well as developing appropriate social skills. Family members and group home staff are able to schedule recreational activities as part of the structure of a client's home life or treatment plan. Any recreational activity can be enjoyable, such as going to the mall, the library, attending music concerts, going out for dinner, going for coffee and going to peer meetings. Peer meeting places occur in the community. Agencies that sponsor these meetings usually have a way of publicizing these events. There are many organizations that sponsor events for the mentally ill in communities. For example the "Drop-In Center" is sponsored by a mental health agency in a nearby town that is convenient to other group homes or client residences. Agencies sometimes advertise in the local newspaper or a family member can contact them to find out when and where recreational activities occur. Some agencies provide bulletins or newsletters about events and some even provide transportation.

Transportation

Transportation arrangements are necessary for medical and recreational activities. They include doctor visits, non-psychiatric medical appointments, appointments for blood tests, attendance at day program, peer meetings and other recreational events.

It is a function of group homes to arrange for transportation for clients. Agencies exist that are in the business of providing transportation for medical and non-medical appointments and the fees can be paid through state-funded medical insurance. For example, a local transport company picks up clients for traveling to a day program site and returns them home in the afternoon. Anyone who has state-funded medical benefits can make appointments for transport on a daily basis with such an agency. This can ease the burden of transportation on family members. Some agencies that sponsor peer events also provide transportation. For example a trip to a local mental health peer dinner night may include a small fee to cover the cost of the dinner and the transportation.

Spiritual and Philosophical support

It is easier for a family member to assist with spiritual needs because it is likely that the family participates in them on a routine basis. Family members can arrange with group home staff to transport clients to meeting places as part of their treatment plan structure. Spiritual and philosophical needs can often be overlooked in group home care. Higher functioning clients can make their needs known to staff and arrangements to attend spiritual or philosophical organizations are possible. These organizations include Christian, Jew, Hindu, Muslim, Universal-Unitarian, Buddhist, and other Higher-Power-based gatherings such as Alcoholics Anonymous or Narcotics Anonymous meetings. Atheist and Agnostic groups are less common in communities but are sometimes listed in phone books.

Many communities are rich in mental health resources. These organizations often publish pamphlets, directories and newsletters and appear in newspaper listings. One only need to make a few phone calls to find out what groups are actively available to your family member or client.

9. Goals and Objectives

Agencies that operate group homes and behavioral health day programs use Treatment Plans to assist clients in learning to live more independently and take care of themselves with less assistance. It would be helpful for family care-givers to be aware of how treatment planning can assist them in caring for their family member. An awareness of a client's treatment plan can assist care-givers in helping clients work toward already existing treatment goals and objectives at a day program or a group home. Therefore, this section contains a very brief description of how goals and objectives within treatment plans are applied, thus serving the purpose of making family care-givers aware of this method.

Goals are increases, reductions, and sustainment of behaviors. Objectives are tasks that contribute to obtaining the goals. Goals are the targets and objectives are the tasks that lead to accomplishing the target. Objectives are measurable. For example, a goal can be to reduce weight and the objective would be eating one less carbohydrate meal per day. An example of a goal might be to increase independent living skills. Its objective would be to obtain and maintain working at a job for a measured period of time or going back to college, taking one or two courses per semester. A psychiatric goal might be to reduce hallucinations, and its objective for accomplishing that goal would be to take medication as prescribed once or twice per day, if necessary. A less abstract goal would be to increase daily living skills, with an objective of cooking at least one meal per day. Ideally, the therapist, social worker or counselor creates a Treatment Plan consisting of goals and objectives for clients. A family care-giver can use a similar approach to help clients reduce irrational or unrealistic thinking, learn specific or "concrete" tasks, determine needs or life skills for survival and comfort, and develop self-awareness. A clinician's Treatment Plan or a family care-giver's plan of action gives the client a structured environment and a clear focus on attaining goals within their physical, social and emotional environments.

Not all goals and objectives are attainable by all clients. A schizophrenic client may not be able to hold their attention span very long or focus on thoughts for anything more than a few seconds. Not all clients are able to exercise in order to lose weight. Not all clients can safely operate a stove or washing machine. In cases where goals and objectives cannot be accomplished, they need to be modified to meet the client's level of functioning. When goals and objectives are not useable, then different, simplified goals and objectives should be targeted. Sometimes staff may be required to assist clients with accomplishing objectives. Helping a client operate a home appliance is part of what is known as "direct care" or "personal care" and is part of the job description of group home counselors.

What Can Happen If You Don't—Critical Thinking Skills Exercise

It takes good organizational skills to be able to assist someone or to be able to adapt to many short or long-term goals and objectives. If the individual does not follow a structured schedule of responsibilities, and if basic needs, such as those described in Section 8 above, are not met, relapse or the return of symptoms, complications and physical, emotional or social problems may develop. Relapse is often referred to as "decompensation" in clinical language. It means that the client's behavior is reverting back to lower-functioning status and symptoms of their diagnosis are returning. Decompensation can happen slowly, over a period of weeks, or quickly, within a day or so, depending on the individual. After decompensation and the return of symptoms the client will need to return to the hospital environment for medication adjustment and stabilization. Often the client's behavior during decompensating will get them in trouble in the community or at their day program. For example, a client may pick up a chair to throw at someone, but may be convinced to put it down. That act could be considered attempted assault and police can be called and the client may either be arrested or taken to a hospital for psychiatric screening. In any case, if a client is determined to be a danger to themself or others then the hospital has the authority to commit them to the psychiatric ward for treatment. The return to a hospital setting in this case is involuntary. An example of voluntary admittance would be if a client is experiencing severe mood swings, extremely active and nervous one day, then feeling very depressed and lethargic the next day and requests being admitted to the hospital for evaluation. The hospital might decide to keep the client for observation during the next day as part of the evaluation. If admitted, the client could be deemed to have a voluntary commitment. Often, clients are not aware of returning symptoms and it is the care-givers or counselors who are able to recognize returning and disturbing, or dangerous, behaviors. Clients who stop taking their medications whenever they feel good are taking the chance of becoming "revolving door" clients by building a history of frequent hospital stays. The hospital staff may get to know them well because of their frequent admissions.

The hospital will keep a client until they are able to function with compliance on the ward. That includes going to activities, talking with counselors, nurses, and doctors about their experience, taking medications and showing average sleeping and eating habits. In general, clients need to show that they are capable of doing what it takes to stay healthy and reduce symptoms. If they are not capable of returning to the community, they will be evaluated for admission to a state psychiatric hospital for long-term care. They may stay in a state hospital for months or years before receiving another attempt at living in the community. During that time new medications will become available that might enable a client to reduce or eliminate symptoms and make a return attempt at living in the community.

Developmental Stages of Recovery

Stage IV: The Client Accepts Long-Term Life Issues of Recovery from Mental Illness

10. Identity

You now realize that you have a mental illness that needs on-going treatment. That means that your daily life activities must change in order for you to stay well. Thoughts about yourself need to change in order for you to adapt to treatment requirements. You may not be able to do some of the things you have been doing in the past as you accept changes in your life. Identity is your perception of yourself and your self-awareness. Accepting your new identity means accepting your new role as a consumer of mental health services, as a psychiatric patient and a client that relies on a mental health agency for care and management of your illness. Examples of mental health agencies are a group home or a day program that you attend. You need to become comfortable with talking about your illness and symptoms to a doctor and to counselors. Here are some things to remember about yourself that can affect your progress and may help you to think positively about moving ahead.

1. We all have done things that we may regret. Begin to accept changes in the here and now. Now is the time of change for the future.

2. You are not the only one. Millions of people have mental illness and are cared for by agencies and family members. If you have no family, remember that the agencies you work with are carefully trying to help you prevent relapse, work toward independent living and return to functioning in the community. The community includes your peers, or others who have mental illness who you can turn to for ideas about achieving goals.

3. You can do something about your illness. You can comply with your treatment plan and learn how to live everyday with the help of your counselors and your psychiatrist.

4. You can change for the better. You are able to complete the tasks that you are given. You can take medication daily for your own well-being. You can accept the care of your family or agency staff. You can accept the idea that they are trying to help you regain activities that you enjoy while maintaining a safe environment for you to live in.

5. You have choices and options. You can decide about how and where to live. Your family may consider having you apply to a group home if living at home does not provide the care you need. You can decide whether or not to participate in recreational activities. You may be able to choose to attend a day program five days a week, or you may request partial attendance of maybe three or four days a week. You may have a choice of day programs. If you don't like one you may be able to try another. You can choose to learn more about your illness by reading books or watching videos about it. You can choose to go to an adult school or go back to college. You can choose to attend AA or NA meetings as part of your treatment plan. You can make choices for participation in the community that follow the goals and objectives of your treatment plan.

Your behavior indicates your intentions. It is not what you say, but what you do that counts. You may have great intentions but your behaviors need to follow your words. Think before doing, and then follow through with action. If your behavior follows your intentions, those around you will be convinced that you are capable of completing the tasks you have decided upon for yourself. Others will come to respect you as a person who is able to get things done. You also need to realize the times when you are not able to complete what you thought you could. We are not always able to complete our goals and objectives. That goes for anyone, not just those who are ill. Some dreams will never be realized and we need to work within our means. That is just part of life. We cannot do it all. Sometimes we have to sacrifice freedom for safety.

6. Helping others can help you also. You can share with others your completion of objectives. You can talk with your peers about what you have accomplished and give them hope for accomplishing things for themselves. Your peers may support you by asking you how things are

going. This allows you to reconsider your thoughts and actions to make sure that you are staying on track and not falling behind the schedule you set for yourself. In turn you can support your peers by providing them with information about the things you have learned and how it feels to succeed at the things you set out to do. Peer support is helpful to others and it can help you to feel confidant that you have made the right choices, can safely carry out your plans and can make progress in your goals and objectives. Writing this book is helping me to remember what I have accomplished in the past, to put my thoughts into action, to plan for the future and to think realistically about what I can or cannot get done. In turn, it may help others to focus on their own thoughts and actions and how they can make progress with the resources and within the environment they live in.

11. Education

You can educate yourself about your illness and about the community and the world. There are two types of education, formal and informal. Formal education means going to accredited schools in the community. It may be something you have been thinking about that you want to put into action. Going back to college is something that requires you to take on new responsibilities yourself. Those responsibilities include applying to the school, arranging finances and transportation. If you are living with your family, you can make phone calls and get the transportation you need, for applying to school and obtaining books and school supplies. If you are living in a group home, you can work with your case manager or one-to-one counselor on completing the tasks needed to prepare for school. You may be eligible for a state or federal grant, which will pay for some or all of your tuition. You will also need time to complete assignments and may need transportation at other times to complete assignments, such as trips to the school library or to other sites for observation. There may be class trips to attend. You will need to learn time management in order to complete your course work. You may need a computer to go to school, or you may need to use computers at the school itself and additional skills may be needed. You may only be able to attend one or two classes a week due to limits on transportation. Being limited does not mean it is impossible. The sooner you start, the sooner you can complete your goal. You need to work with your family or counselors in order to gain their help and cooperation with going to school. Attending college helps you to learn more about the world today and the community in which you live. It is therefore an aid to returning to the community, which is part of your treatment plan.

Informal education is available to most consumers. Many day program and group home agencies provide counseling groups that discuss with and inform clients about medication, symptoms of mental illness, chemical addiction, and diet and nutrition. Aside from these groups, you may be able to attend adult school classes during the week that are available through the community. You may be able to take a course in using a computer, perhaps a course in health care or a recreational course, such as drawing, or crafting. This type of education also helps you to become aware of community resources that are available to you, such as the library computer for exploring the internet, or activities held at your local Mental Health Association.

The National Mental Health Association website has all of the latest information about mental health issues. The address is www.nmha.org. There may be a National Mental Health Association affiliate office in your county, which will have much reading material regarding clinical treatment planning and consumer needs and methods of working toward higher functioning in the community.

12. Stigma Awareness

Stigma is the belief held by others that people with mental illness or other disabilities are not capable of staying well or completing life tasks and will always be a disruption or problem to the community and the people they are in contact with. It is a negative connotation which is prejudice and discrimination. Stigma may cause others to deliberately avoid contact with the mentally ill and disabled. Stigma exists largely because of news stories about mental health patients becoming violent, along with stereotyping in the media.

There are many myths about people with mental illness, for example, people with mental illness can never be normal, people with mental illness can not hold important positions, persons with mental illness are dangerous. The person with mental illness needs to be aware that disclosing about their illness may result in a stigmatic reaction from others. The National Mental Health Association suggests that sharing your experience with mental illness and showing that mental illness is nothing to be embarrassed about can help reduce stigma. The NMHA has a fact sheet available about stigma at www.nmha.org. A person with mental illness pursuing an education in psychology, social work or counseling can learn ways of advocating for the mentally ill and explore ways of reducing stigma in their community for themself and others.

13. Resources of Information

Information and education about mental illness, treatment and family member support is not always easy to obtain. You won't find many supporting agencies, groups or social activities in the phone book. This is because many agencies that provide activities and education for clients and family members are part of larger agencies or facilities. For example, a Social Club is sponsored and run by the county office of the National Mental Health Association. Information would be available only from that office about Social Club meeting times and events. Here is another example: A local hospital offers a medication education group that meets every week for client support and information about coping with medication. A client would have to contact the hospital for the phone number for the group leader and to join the group. Below are some suggestions for finding support services in your community.

Local Newspapers

Some self-help meeting and activity groups will report their events to the local newspapers for print in the Community Events section of the paper (usually in the back pages.) This is a start. Calling these phone numbers may provide access to other groups and phone numbers. All you have to do is ask. Many of these groups are free, may be covered by state insurance or may be available at very low cost.

College or Universities

Going to college to learn about the mental health system is the most educational thing you can do. It takes good time management skills, places to be quiet for study, a computer, and a strong will to succeed. However, if you are not ready to make such a commitment you can use the local college library for information. Most college libraries are open to the public. You would need to apply for a library card and observe the rules of the library for the general public. It is very likely that you will find books about the types of mental illness, managing mental illness, and clinical treatment techniques. You may also find books written by others with mental illness.

Hospitals

You may find some social service organizations in the phone book under "Social Services," however not all non-profit agencies will be willing to pay for this kind of advertising. The best way to find local non-profit agencies is to call hospitals and ask if there are any local outside agencies that provide a service you need. You may have to start by asking for Outpatient Mental Health Services, who then may direct you to a social worker or a person who provides information to clients about local agencies and the services they provide, such as meetings, therapy groups or other activities.

Local Non-Profit Agencies

Many non-profit organizations publish newsletters and pamphlets about groups and social activities for mental health clients which they provide. Some agencies share information about other agencies for services that they do not provide. For example one agency owns and operates the Drop-In Center, a building where local clients can gather to meet peers several times per week. That agency will call other agencies to invite them to use the Drop-In Center and provide them with the times of service. The service costs nothing. The participating agency needs only to provide transportation to the center. Calling agencies to inquire about services they provide may also lead you to more phone numbers, other agencies and more free or low-cost services.

The National Mental Health Association

The internet available at your local library provides almost all of the basic information about mental illness from the National Mental Health Association. The website is www.nmha.org. Spending time reading features on the site, taking notes, or printing out articles can be very empowering. The information on this site can help you to learn better self-care and give you ideas for therapeutic activities in which you may want to try (if available in your community). There will also be links to other websites for even more information.

There is a bonus to using the NMHA. Some larger counties in your state may have a county office of the NMHA. That office provides a great deal of information about mental illness, treatment and even recovery. They may provide a library and reading area for you. All you need is the transportation to reach an extraordinary amount of free information about mental health issues. You can call Outpatient Services at hospitals or a local non-profit agency who may be able to provide you with the number of the National Mental Health Association in your area. Whatever your topic, it will probably be available at the NMHA library.

The National Alliance on Mental Health, or NAMI is an organization dedicated to providing information about mental health issues to its members and the public. Its website can be reached at www.nami.org.

Psychiatrist

The psychiatrist is the authority on medication. Meetings with psychiatrists are brief, ranging from 10 minutes to 30 minutes, usually. In order to have your questions answered, keep a list of questions about your medication and its effects. Bring the list to your next psychiatric consultation and you will be prepared to make the most of the time spent with the doctor. Some ideas for questions are: old versus new medicines, taking meds at night to reduce drowsiness during the day, side effects that prevent you from daily activities, such as blurred vision or extreme dizziness. The practice of keeping a list of medical questions may also be useful for meetings with your general practitioner.

Pharmacy

The pharmacy is a secondary source of medical information. In addition to providing print outs about the medications you take, the pharmacy may carry some helpful books, such as *The Pill Book*, which lists and describes almost every brand of medication, its use, and includes side effects. Larger chain drug stores sell a variety of books about medical care. Remember to discuss changes in your treatment with your psychiatrist first. Without your psychiatric medication in place, you run the risk of losing all of the ground you have gained in your recovery.

LaVergne, TN USA
19 November 2009
164651LV00004B/122/A